SELENIUM FOR BEGINNERS

Unlocking Vital Health With Selenium, A Comprehensive Guide To Boosting Immunity, Preventing Diseases, And Enhancing Well-Being

Georgette Lockett

DISCLAIMER

The author of this book is not affiliated, associated, endorsed, sponsored, or approved by any company or individual. The views and opinions expressed in this book are solely those of the author and do not necessarily reflect the official policy or position of any entity.

The author hereby disclaims any relationship, collaboration, or partnership with any company or individual mentioned in this book. Any references to products, services, or individuals are provided for informational purposes only and should not be construed as an endorsement or recommendation.

Readers are advised to exercise their own judgment and discretion when applying the information provided in this book. The author shall not be held responsible for any actions taken by readers based on the content of this book.

This book is intended for general informational purposes only, and the author makes no representations or warranties of any kind, express or implied, about the completeness, accuracy, reliability, suitability, or availability of the information contained herein. Any reliance on the information in this book is at the reader's own risk.

The author reserves the right to update, change, or modify any information in this book without notice. It is the responsibility of the reader to verify any information before taking any actions based on the content of this book.

By reading this book, the reader acknowledges and agrees to the terms of this disclaimer.

Table of Contents

INTRODUCTION

Selenium, a trace element, is essential for preserving human health. This tutorial seeks to give a thorough knowledge of Selenium, highlighting its significance and providing insights into its numerous aspects. By the conclusion of this investigation, readers will have a better understanding of the function Selenium plays in fostering well-being.

Brief Overview Of Selenium

Selenium, denoted by the molecular symbol Se, is a necessary micronutrient for both humans and animals. Its biological relevance was originally discovered in the late 1950s, and substantial study has since underlined its varied benefits to health.

Importance Of Selenium In Human Health

Selenium is essential for many physiological functions, functioning as a cofactor for selenoproteins, a protein class that contains Selenium in the form of the amino acid selenocysteine. Selenoproteins play roles in antioxidant defense, thyroid hormone metabolism, DNA synthesis, and immunological function. Selenium's high antioxidant qualities make it an important participant in the body's neutralization of damaging free radicals, lowering oxidative stress.

Purpose And Structure Of The Guide

This article is designed to give a thorough examination of Selenium, including its many functions and effects on human health. Each section digs into a different element of Selenium, from its activities in the body to dietary sources and possible health consequences. Readers may easily traverse the book by grouping the content into discrete chapters, acquiring a comprehensive grasp of Selenium.

CHAPTER 1

What Is Selenium?

Selenium is an important trace element that plays an important part in many physiological processes that are needed for human health. This chapter goes into the definition, characteristics, natural sources, and chemical properties of Selenium to provide a thorough knowledge of its relevance.

Definition And Characteristics

Selenium, with the chemical symbol Se, is a trace element in the periodic table's chalcogen group. It has features that put it in the same category as sulfur, tellurium, and polonium. Selenium, discovered in 1817, has subsequently been recognized for its biological significance.

Selenium is unusual in that it can be incorporated into amino acids to generate selenoproteins. These selenoproteins are required for the normal operation of a variety of biological functions, including antioxidant defense and thyroid hormone metabolism.

Natural Sources Of Selenium

Understanding Selenium's natural sources is critical for maintaining proper levels in the body. Brazil nuts, seafood (such as tuna and shrimp), chicken, eggs, dairy products, and whole grains are all high in selenium. The concentration of Selenium in soil has a substantial impact on its abundance in plant-based meals, highlighting the necessity of taking regional differences in dietary consumption into account.

Chemical Properties And Forms

Selenium has a wide range of chemical characteristics and exists in a variety of oxidation states. Selenide, selenite, and selenate are the most prevalent types.

These various forms influence Selenium's bioavailability and biological activity inside the body.

Selenoproteins, which include the amino acid selenocysteine, play an important role in Selenium's biological activity. Selenoproteins that contribute to antioxidant defense, redox control, and thyroid hormone metabolism include glutathione peroxidases, thioredoxin reductases, and iodothyronine deiodinases.

Understanding Selenium's chemical forms is critical for determining its dietary intake and associated health benefits. Its proper usage inside the body is ensured by the balance of its many forms.

Finally, this chapter introduces the element selenium, including its description, features, natural sources, and chemical properties. As we go through the chapters, we will look at the many functions of selenium in human health, highlighting its importance in general well-being.

CHAPTER 2

Functions And Benefits Of Selenium

Selenium, an important trace mineral, is necessary for human health owing to its many roles inside the body. Its diverse contributions span several systems and processes, demonstrating its importance in overall well-being.

Role Of Selenium In The Body

One of the most important activities of selenium is as a cofactor for numerous enzymes, notably selenoproteins, which are required for proper physiological processes. Selenoproteins that serve as antioxidants, such as glutathione peroxidases and thioredoxin reductases, protect cells from oxidative stress by neutralizing damaging free radicals. Because of its function in preventing oxidative damage, selenium is essential for cellular health and lifespan.

Antioxidant Properties

The antioxidant properties of selenium are notable. To battle oxidative stress and prevent cellular damage, it acts in conjunction with other antioxidants such as vitamins C and E. This characteristic not only helps to preserve skin health, but it also helps the immune system by protecting immune cells from oxidative damage and therefore keeping their effectiveness.

Contribution To Immune Function And Thyroid Health

Selenium has a complex relationship with immunological function. Adequate amounts of selenium are linked to a healthy immunological response. Selenoproteins aid in the regulation of immunological responses and inflammatory processes, enhancing the body's capacity to fight infections and disorders.

Furthermore, selenium is essential for thyroid function. It is an essential component in the production of thyroid hormones. The thyroid gland has the highest concentration of selenium per gram of tissue of any organ in the body, highlighting the mineral's relevance in thyroid function. Selenium assists in the conversion of inactive thyroid hormone (T4) to active thyroid hormone (T3). This conversion mechanism is critical for controlling metabolism, development, and energy levels in general.

Understanding selenium's varied functions elucidates its importance to human health. Selenium is an essential mineral due to its antioxidant qualities that fight cellular damage as well as its critical role in immunological function and thyroid health. A lack of selenium may cause a variety of health problems, underlining the necessity of getting enough via food or supplementation.

By recognizing and respecting selenium's many roles, one may better understand its importance in sustaining good health. The following sections will go further into the sources, dietary recommendations, and possible hazards linked with selenium, to provide a thorough guide for reaping its advantages.

CHAPTER 3

Selenium Deficiency

Selenium, a trace element that is important for human health, is involved in a variety of physiological functions. Understanding selenium insufficiency is critical, since low levels may cause a variety of health problems. The origins, symptoms, and groups at risk of selenium insufficiency are discussed in this chapter.

Causes And Risk Factors

Selenium insufficiency is caused by several circumstances. Soil composition has a considerable impact on plant selenium concentration, hence impacting crop selenium levels. Low soil selenium levels may result in foods with inadequate selenium, resulting in a deficit in the local population. Furthermore, industrial pollution and some agricultural methods may deplete soil selenium, worsening the situation.

Dietary choices also influence selenium intake. Individuals who follow strict diets or consume foods cultivated in selenium-deficient regions may not get enough selenium. Furthermore, illnesses such as Crohn's disease or other malabsorption disorders might impair the body's capacity to absorb and use selenium properly, raising the risk of shortage.

Symptoms And Health Implications

Recognizing the signs of selenium insufficiency is critical for prompt treatment. Selenium is required for selenoproteins to function as antioxidants, protecting cells from oxidative stress. Without enough selenium, the body's capacity to neutralize free radicals declines, possibly resulting in cellular damage.

Fatigue, muscular weakness, and impaired immune function are common indications of selenium insufficiency. More severe signs, such as joint discomfort, hair loss, and reproductive difficulties, may arise over time. Notably, a lack of selenium has been related to an increased risk of various ailments, including cardiovascular disease and some forms of cancer.

Populations At Risk Of Deficiency

Because of lifestyle, dietary choices, or physiological reasons, some populations are more vulnerable to selenium deficiency. If vegetarians and vegans do not eat selenium-rich animal products, their selenium intake may be decreased. Residents of selenium-deficient soil areas, notably in portions of China, Eastern Europe, and New Zealand, are at a higher risk of insufficiency.

Pregnant and lactating women need more selenium for fetal development and nursing, making them more prone to insufficiency if their food intake is insufficient. The elderly may also be at risk owing to decreased absorption and possible dietary restrictions.

Finally, knowing the origins, symptoms, and groups at risk of selenium insufficiency is critical for general health promotion. To address the selenium shortage, interventions such as dietary diversity, selenium supplementation if needed, and raising awareness of the relevance of this trace element in maintaining optimum well-being must be implemented. Individuals may contribute to a healthier and more resilient population by detecting and reducing selenium deficiency.

CHAPTER 4

Selenium Toxicity

Selenium, a trace mineral that is essential for health, acts in a restricted range where its advantages are most visible. However, exceeding the prescribed amounts might have major health consequences. Understanding selenium poisoning, including its causes, symptoms, and acceptable limits, is critical for sustaining good health.

Sources Of Excessive Selenium Intake

Selenium toxicity is most often caused by excessive intake, which may occur via dietary supplements or inadvertent absorption from environmental sources. Regions with high soil selenium concentration may farm crops with high selenium levels, leading to overexposure.

Supplements, although healthy in moderation, may be harmful if eaten in excess. Many multivitamins and mineral supplements include selenium, which might result in an unintended overdose when combined with other selenium-rich meals.

Symptoms And Health Risks Associated With Overdose

The symptoms of selenium poisoning may vary in severity, from moderate to severe. Early symptoms may include gastrointestinal difficulties such as nausea and diarrhea, as well as brittle hair and nails. Chronic selenium exposure may result in selenosis, a disorder marked by more severe symptoms such as neurological problems, skin lesions, and a garlic-like stench in the breath.

Long-term selenium overexposure may have a harmful influence on general health. Its buildup in tissues may harm organs, particularly the kidneys and liver. Furthermore, too much selenium may upset the body's antioxidant equilibrium, resulting in oxidative stress and probable cell damage.

Recommended Upper Limits

To reduce the hazards of selenium intoxication, regulatory authorities across the globe have set suggested maximum limits for daily consumption. The tolerated upper intake limit (UL) for adults is commonly established at 400-450 mcg per day, with regional standards differing somewhat.

Although pregnant and lactating women need somewhat more selenium, excessive doses may be hazardous to both the mother and the growing baby. The suggested limits for children are substantially lower, reflecting their smaller body size and distinct metabolic demands.

It is crucial to follow these instructions to avoid selenium poisoning. To maintain acceptable levels, selenium consumption from both food sources and supplementation must be monitored. It is best to consult with a healthcare practitioner before beginning any new supplement regimen, especially if you live in an area with naturally high selenium levels in the soil or water.

Understanding the delicate balance of selenium consumption is critical for reaping the advantages while avoiding the negative consequences of overexposure. Responsible intake and knowledge of sources may protect against the hazards of selenium poisoning, enabling people to improve their health without jeopardizing their well-being.

CHAPTER 5

Selenium In Human Nutrition

Selenium, an important trace mineral, plays a critical function in human health maintenance. Understanding its recommended dietary allowances (RDAs) and the intricacies of supplementation is critical for maintaining appropriate bodily balance.

Recommended Dietary Allowances (RDAs)

The required selenium consumption varies according to age, gender, and life stage. Adults need around 55 micrograms per day. This figure may change significantly depending on conditions such as pregnancy or breastfeeding. Selenium-rich foods, such as Brazil nuts, fish, chicken, and cereals, may help considerably achieve these needs.

Selenium Supplementation: Pros And Cons

Individuals with low food intake or who live in areas with selenium-deficient soils may benefit from supplementation. However, supplementing must be approached with caution.

Pros

- **Addressing Deficiency:** Supplements may help people who live in areas with low soil selenium levels by decreasing deficiency concerns.

- **Specific Health issues:** In certain situations, selenium supplementation may help with the management of specific health issues, such as thyroid abnormalities or immune function support.

Cons

- **Potential Toxicity:** Selenium toxicity is a worry since excessive ingestion may cause selenosis, which is characterized by symptoms such as hair loss, brittle nails, and digestive difficulties.

• **Interaction with Other Nutrients:** Selenium interacts with other nutrients; excessive use may upset the balance, thereby compromising general health.

Balancing Selenium Intake For Optimal Health

A balanced selenium consumption requires a careful approach. Here are a few ideas:

Diversification of Diet: Eating a diverse diet rich in selenium-containing foods helps provide a natural and balanced intake.

Consultation with Healthcare Providers: Anyone thinking about taking selenium should talk to their doctor. They may provide tailored advice depending on an individual's health situation, assuring safe and effective supplementing.

Monitoring Selenium Levels: Regular monitoring of selenium levels via medical testing might help guide proper dietary changes or supplement use.

Environmental Awareness: Geographical location, soil type, and agricultural techniques all impact selenium concentration in food. Understanding these factors may help people make more educated food decisions.

To achieve appropriate selenium levels, a balanced strategy that combines a diversified diet rich in selenium sources with judicious supplementation, when necessary, under expert supervision is required. Striking this equilibrium may improve general health while reducing the hazards associated with lack or overuse of this vital mineral.

CHAPTER 6

Selenium And Disease Prevention

Selenium, a trace element, is important in disease prevention and contributes to many areas of human health. This chapter delves into the delicate relationship between selenium and chronic disease prevention, offering light on its influence on cancer and cardiovascular health.

Selenium's Role In Preventing Chronic Diseases

Selenium's antioxidant qualities make it a strong force in the body's fight against damaging free radicals. As a result, selenium protects cells against oxidative stress, which is a major contributor to chronic illnesses. Furthermore, selenium is required for the formation of selenoproteins, which are enzymes with a variety of activities. These selenoproteins play important roles in cellular processes such as immunological response, DNA synthesis, and thyroid hormone metabolism.

Relationship Between Selenium And Cancer

One of the most studied areas of selenium's health effect is its possible involvement in cancer prevention. Selenium has been linked to a lower risk of some malignancies by functioning as an antioxidant and anti-inflammatory agent.

According to research, appropriate selenium levels in the body may help to prevent the development of malignancies such as lung, colon, prostate, and breast cancer. However, the association between selenium and cancer is complicated, and ideal levels are critical since both lack and excess may be harmful.

Cardiovascular Health And Selenium

The impact of selenium goes beyond cancer prevention to cardiovascular health. Selenium is an essential component of antioxidant enzymes, which help to protect the heart and blood vessels from oxidative stress. It promotes blood vessel flexibility and decreases inflammation, resulting in a healthier cardiovascular system. Adequate selenium levels have been linked to a decreased risk of cardiovascular illnesses such as heart attacks and strokes.

Understanding the complicated relationship between selenium and disease prevention stresses the need to maintain appropriate selenium levels for general health. It is important to remember, however, that the effects of selenium are subtle, and individual reactions may differ.

As with any vitamin, finding the proper balance is critical. While selenium is essential for health, too much of it may be hazardous. As a result, a well-balanced diet high in selenium-containing foods such as Brazil nuts, fish, chicken, and whole grains is advised. Additionally, where required, consulting with healthcare specialists may give tailored advice on selenium supplementation.

Finally, the link between selenium and illness prevention emphasizes the importance of this trace mineral in sustaining good health. From countering oxidative stress to aiding in cancer prevention and cardiovascular health, selenium is an essential component in the complex web of human biology. As research into the complexity of this critical element continues, including selenium in a balanced lifestyle remains an important facet of improving long-term health and disease resiliency.

CHAPTER 7

Selenium In Agriculture And Environment

Selenium, a trace element vital for human health, is important not only for our health but also for agriculture and the environment. This chapter delves into the complex interaction between selenium and soil, as well as the ramifications for agricultural productivity and ecological sustainability.

Selenium In Soil And Its Impact On Food Crops

Selenium's trip starts in the soil, where its availability has a considerable impact on plant selenium concentration. Globally, the content of selenium in soil fluctuates, resulting in places with selenium-rich or selenium-deficient soils.

Plants take selenium from the soil and store it in their tissues, allowing it to enter the food chain.

Understanding selenium levels in soil is critical for agriculture since it directly influences crop nutritional quality. Selenium-rich soil increases crop selenium content, providing an important nutritional supply for both animals and humans. Conversely, selenium-deficient soil may result in crops with insufficient selenium levels, causing problems for places with low natural selenium availability.

Environmental Concerns And Selenium Toxicity In Ecosystems

While selenium is necessary in tiny quantities, excessive amounts may be harmful to both terrestrial and aquatic environments. Selenium poisoning is an issue in locations where natural deposits or human activity raise selenium levels in the environment.

High selenium levels may damage plants, animals, and microbes, causing ecological equilibrium to be disrupted.

Aquatic habitats, in particular, are in danger from selenium pollution. Selenium may build up in bodies of water, causing harm to fish and other aquatic animals. Understanding and addressing these environmental challenges is critical for sustaining biodiversity and ecosystem health.

Regulations And Management Strategies

Because selenium is both a crucial nutrient and a possible environmental danger, regulatory measures and management techniques are critical. Authorities throughout the globe have set recommendations for monitoring selenium levels in soil, water, and food items, to strike a balance between protecting human health and protecting the environment.

Sustainable agricultural methods, such as soil amendments to increase selenium content and reduce inadequacies, are part of effective management strategies. Selenium must also be considered in wastewater treatment and industrial operations to avoid uncontrolled emissions into the environment.

As we navigate the intricate web of selenium's impact on agriculture and the environment, it becomes clear that responsible management practices are critical to maximizing benefits while mitigating risks. Balancing the delicate balance between selenium's functions in human health and its environmental implications is critical for a healthy and sustainable future.

CHAPTER 8

Selenium In Research And Medical Applications

Selenium, a trace element essential for human health, has received a great deal of interest in scientific study and medicinal applications owing to its diverse qualities. Ongoing research continues to uncover its potential medicinal applications, expanding its reach beyond nutritional value.

Current Scientific Studies And Ongoing Research

Modern scientific research is delving into the various mechanics of selenium's effect inside the body. Researchers are interested in its role as an essential micronutrient, as well as its bioavailability, metabolism, and interactions with other nutrients. Studies are being conducted to investigate the relationship between selenium consumption and disease prevention, to determine optimum daily intake amounts for specific groups.

Emerging research fields look at the molecular mechanisms that selenium uses to produce its antioxidative properties. Investigations are being conducted into its role in gene expression, cell signaling, and its ability to modulate immune responses. Advanced approaches such as metabolomics and proteomics assist in understanding the role of selenium in biological systems at the molecular level.

Potential Therapeutic Uses And Applications

The versatility of selenium has sparked interest in potential therapeutic applications in a variety of medical domains. Because of its antioxidant properties, it is an appealing candidate for treating oxidative stress-related conditions. Selenium's role in thyroid function has prompted research into its use in treating thyroid disorders such as autoimmune thyroiditis.

Furthermore, because of selenium's intriguing role in immune function regulation, researchers are looking into its potential implications for autoimmune diseases. Preliminary research indicates that selenium has a promising role in modulating inflammatory responses, potentially opening the door to therapeutic interventions in conditions such as rheumatoid arthritis and inflammatory bowel disease.

Selenium In Medicine And Healthcare

Selenium has applications in healthcare and medicine in addition to its traditional role as a dietary supplement. Selenium compounds have been studied for their potential use in cancer therapy, particularly in enhancing the effects of standard treatments such as chemotherapy and radiation. More clinical trials, however, are required to validate these findings and determine their efficacy and safety.

Furthermore, the importance of selenium in reproductive health has gotten attention, with studies looking into its role in fertility and pregnancy-related complications. Studies on the effect of selenium supplementation on male and female fertility offer promising avenues for future interventions.

The growing field of nanotechnology has increased interest in selenium nanoparticles. Because of their potential for enhanced bioavailability and reduced toxicity, these nanoparticles are being investigated for targeted drug delivery systems and various biomedical applications.

Finally, ongoing research continues to reveal the many facets of selenium, demonstrating its potential beyond basic nutrition. Its multifunctional properties and promising therapeutic applications highlight the importance of further investigation, presenting opportunities for innovative medical interventions and healthcare advancements.

CHAPTER 9

Dietary Sources Of Selenium

Selenium, an important micronutrient, is required for a variety of physiological functions in the human body. While Selenium is only required in trace quantities by the human body, its importance in general health cannot be emphasized. Getting Selenium from food is essential for maintaining optimum levels and supporting good health.

Natural Food Sources Rich In Selenium

Selenium may be present in a wide range of foods. This vital element is plentiful in seafood, notably fish and shellfish such as tuna, sardines, shrimp, and salmon. Furthermore, nuts such as Brazil nuts are one of the finest natural sources of selenium. Other nuts, such as walnuts and sunflower seeds, contain selenium in lesser levels.

Selenium is abundant in poultry, including chicken and turkey, as well as meats such as beef and lamb. Grains and cereals may contribute to Selenium consumption at variable levels depending on the soil composition in which they grow. Selenium is also found in vegetables, including spinach, broccoli, and garlic.

Recommended Dietary Habits To Maintain Adequate Levels

A balanced diet is essential for ensuring enough Selenium consumption. A varied diet that includes a number of the aforementioned items may assist in achieving optimal Selenium levels. The Selenium content of food, on the other hand, is strongly dependent on the soil in which it is cultivated or the feed supplied to animals, resulting in differences in Selenium levels.

Individuals living in areas with low soil Selenium concentration may find it difficult to meet acceptable levels via food alone. In such instances, contemplating Selenium supplementation under the supervision of a healthcare practitioner may be essential.

Cooking And Processing Effects On Selenium Content

The technique of food preparation might affect Selenium levels. Because of its solubility in water, cooking, particularly boiling and steaming, may reduce selenium levels. However, the degree of the loss is determined by parameters such as cooking temperature and time. Certain cooking techniques, such as roasting or baking, may, on the other hand, keep Selenium content better.

Furthermore, food processing and refining practices might have an impact on Selenium levels. Because the outer layers where Selenium accumulates are removed in refined grains, they contain less Selenium than whole grains.

To summarize, although selenium is accessible in a variety of natural food sources, maintaining optimal intake requires making conscious dietary choices as well as knowing the influence of food processing and cooking techniques. A well-balanced diet rich in Selenium-rich foods is essential for maintaining appropriate Selenium levels for general health and well-being.

CHAPTER 10

Integrating Selenium Into A Healthy Lifestyle

Selenium is a critical micronutrient that is required for a variety of biological activities, making its presence in a well-balanced diet essential for good health. Incorporating Selenium-rich foods and making smart supplementation decisions may greatly improve overall health.

Practical Tips For Incorporating Selenium-Rich Foods

A well-balanced diet is essential for getting enough Selenium. Brazil nuts, seafood (such as tuna, shrimp, and salmon), chicken, eggs, dairy products, and whole grains are all high in selenium. Selenium levels may be increased by including these items in regular meals.

Consider rotating food sources to vary nutritional intake and minimize over-reliance on single things. Brazil nuts, for example, are very high in Selenium and should be taken in moderation owing to their high content.

Considerations For Supplementation

Individuals at risk of Selenium deficiency, such as those living in areas with low soil Selenium levels or those following restricted diets, may need supplementation. However, it is critical to speak with a healthcare practitioner before beginning any supplement program to prevent overdoing it, which may have negative consequences.

When purchasing supplements, go for reputed companies with third-party certifications to assure quality and precise doses. Excessive Selenium supplementation may cause toxicity and other negative health consequences.

Overall Lifestyle Choices For Optimal Selenium Intake

Apart from food choices and supplements, lifestyle modifications might boost Selenium absorption and utilization:

1. **Balanced Diet:** To promote general health and nutritional intake, prioritize a diversified and balanced diet rich in fruits, vegetables, whole grains, and lean meats.

2. **Avoiding Over processing:** Limit your consumption of overly processed foods, which frequently contain fewer nutrients, including Selenium, as a result of refining procedures.

3. **Environmental Awareness:** Learn about the environmental elements that influence selenium concentration in food and its effect on ecosystems. Support long-term farming methods that preserve soil health and nutrient levels.

4. Periodic health checks may uncover any possible deficiencies or imbalances, prompting dietary or supplemental modifications as required.

By taking a comprehensive approach to diet and health, people may guarantee appropriate Selenium intake, supporting critical biological processes and perhaps lowering the risk of numerous health conditions linked with Selenium insufficiency.

Conclusion

In this complete investigation of Selenium, we've spanned its essential core, from its responsibilities inside the body to its influence on the environment, and its critical relevance in preserving health. Selenium, an important micronutrient, bears significant relevance for human health and ecological equilibrium.

Summary Of Key Points Discussed

We started by defining Selenium, offering light on its natural origins and various chemical features. Its vital roles inside the body, such as functioning as an antioxidant powerhouse, boosting immunological function, and contributing considerably to thyroid health, were underlined. Furthermore, we highlighted the crucial ramifications of the Selenium shortage, including the sources, symptoms, and groups especially prone to its insufficiency.

Delving further, we studied the relationship between Selenium and illness prevention. Notably, its promise in battling chronic illnesses like cancer and its good effect on cardiovascular health reflects its substantial impact. Additionally, we explored Selenium's consequences in agriculture and its dual nature—beneficial in ideal amounts for crops, but potentially hazardous when accumulated in excess within ecosystems.

Importance Of Maintaining Balanced Selenium Levels

Maintaining a healthy Selenium intake appears as a key part of health. While its shortage may lead to several health concerns, excessive ingestion might pose environmental hazards. Striking a balance is key—through natural food sources and, where required, educated supplementation under expert advice.

Selenium, frequently classified as a trace mineral, plays a tremendous role in maintaining human functioning and keeping ecological balance. Its multifarious participation in human health, from reinforcing the immune system to possibly preventing chronic illnesses, cannot be stressed. Yet, this voyage into Selenium's complexity also underscores the necessity for a careful approach, realizing that balance is vital for both human health and environmental sustainability.

In conclusion, building an awareness of Selenium's relevance in health and agriculture empowers us to make educated choices—adopting a balanced strategy to ensure its advantages without tipping the scales towards deficiency or excess. Let us embrace this information to nourish our well-being and contribute to a healthy, peaceful planet.

THE END